EASY GUIDES TO COMMON HEALTH TOPICS

SVETLANA PYATIGORSKAYA,
FNP, APRN, ABAAHP

To order additional copies of this book, contact:
Xlibris
844-714-8691
www.Xlibris.com
Orders@Xlibris.com

ISBN: Softcover   978-1-6641-6055-2
        EBook   978-1-6641-6054-5

Print information available on the last page

Rev. date: 05/03/2021

PREFACE

I had not started this work as a book. My first guide had been created as a patient handout about thyroid disease. My need was practical and simple. I see the patients every day in a clinical setting, and every day, I must give an explanation about the same health problems. This experience helped me to identify the gaps in common knowledge typical for many people. It is not easy for a person without a medical background to grasp all information in a time-limiting and highly stressful environment of a doctor's visit. My goal was to create a simple but meaningful guide with essential information that the patient can take home, read without rush, and then plan the changes she or he needs to do to take control over the disease.

I am a nurse practitioner. What it means I am a nurse, and nurses believe in the importance of patient education and empowering people with knowledge.

But in addition to being a family nurse practitioner, I am an American Board of Anti-Aging Health practitioner. I am practicing functional medicine parallel to conventional primary care practice. Well, it is not a parallel, I must admit. It is in conjunction because you cannot switch mindsets just by switching rooms. I could not help including these two views: the conventional and functional medicine concepts in my guide. And when it had happened, I gave my guide to the patients, and they like it. I gave my guide to the colleague, and they like it too. I am being asked to create handouts for several more topics, and I had said yes.

I created a post-Bariatric body guide. I am a gastric bypass survivor, and I am participating in several post-bariatric social media groups. I came across the post from a person who had surgery and now was discharged into the care of her primary care. Post-bariatric care is an area of expertise that required certain knowledge. Not all providers are equally competent at this specific topic. Unfortunately, it did look like the doctor of my social media peer was not very familiar with the topic. I posted an offer in the group, telling them about my guide and offering to email the PDF to anyone who will send me a request. Over the next twenty-four hours, I had emailed several hundreds of guides, and the requests were still coming. Finally, I had to admit that I cannot fulfill the promise to email the guide and created a Dropbox link, allowing me to access anyone who wanted to download it. But experienced was clear: there is a need for my information.

After the bariatric surgery topic, it was natural to speak about obesity and weight loss. And obesity comes side by side with blood glucose metabolic disease. All my guides include information about balancing vitamins and minerals in the diet and the role of deficiencies in the disease's development. Nutritional deficiencies led to a conversation about wellness IV therapy. And now, I had all the topics presented in this volume.

I decided I need to print the guides and made them downloadable from my website. The long story made short, soon I found it just easier to turn the guides into the book, so I did.

I tried my best to include evidence-based information, but I had also filtered it through my own clinical experience and had always had my patients in my mind. I do not have the goal to make an academic essay. I want it to be simple and helpful to anyone. I hope I succeeded, and you will enjoy the book!

EASY GUIDE TO UNDERSTAND YOUR THYROID DISEASE

THE THYROID IS A GLAND IN YOUR NECK. IT PRODUCES THE THYROID HORMONES.

- There are two types of thyroid problems that are possible: structural or functional.

- The structural problems are the changes that may occur with the gland itself. It may get enlarged. It also may develop nodules (a tumor) or cysts (bag filled up with fluids).

- Most often, those changes can be found by your primary care provider during an exam or at the image studies, such as a thyroid sonogram and neck CT.

- Most nodules and cysts are benign, but some may be a cancer. In general, if the nodule or cyst > 1cm in size, it needs to undergo a biopsy to check for cancer cells.

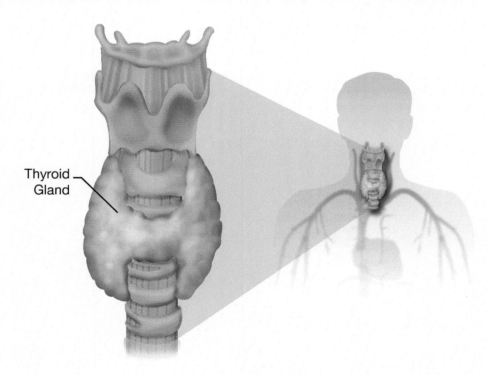

Thyroid Gland

FUNCTIONAL CHANGES OF THE THYROID ARE CHANGES IN THE NUMBER OF THYROID HORMONES PRODUCED BY THE GLAND. THYROID HORMONES REGULATE MANY FUNCTIONS IN OUR BODY: THE CALCIUM IN THE BONES, INVOLVED IN THE ENERGY PRODUCTION OF THE MUSCLES; REGULATE THE FUNCTIONING OF THE REPRODUCTIVE ORGANS; AND REGULATES WEIGHT, HEART RATE, MOOD, AND MENTAL WELL-BEING.

- Too much thyroid hormones is called hyperthyroidism

- **Symptoms associated with hyperthyroidism are the following:**

- Weight loss, increased appetite

- Fast heart rate

- Body swelling

- Anxiety, insomnia

- Cold intolerance

- Hair loss

- Shaking of the body

- Sweating

- Fatigue

- Diarrhea

- Changes in menstrual cycle, infertility, loss of menstruation, and more.

- **Not enough thyroid hormones is called hyperthyroidism**

- **Symptoms associated with hyperthyroidism are the following:**

- Weight gain and difficulty in losing weight

- Slow heart rate

- Swelling around the eyes and ankles

- Depression, anxiety. memory loss

- Cold intolerance, cold hands and feet

- Thinning hair, dry skin

- Intolerance to exercise, fatigue

- Pain in the joints

- Constipation

- Menstrual irregularity, pain, infertility

FUNCTIONAL CHANGES OF THE THYROID CAN BE FOUND THROUGH BLOOD WORK

THERE ARE 5 THYROID HORMONES PRODUCED BY THYROID GLAND: CALCITONIN, T1, T2, T3, AND T4

- Calcitonin acts by decreasing the calcium in the blood and helps to preserve it in the bone.

Eighty percent of the thyroid hormones produced are T4. However, T4 is a storage form of thyroid hormones and cannot be used by the cells. To be used, it needs to be converted into T3.

The remained 20% of thyroid hormones are the combination of T1, T2, and T3.

There is still no comprehensive understanding of the roles of T1 and T2. T2 is known to be important for cellular energy production in the heart, liver, skeletal muscles through an increase of oxygen consumption.

T3 is the active hormone, and all those functions associated with thyroid regulation is primarily carried out by T3.

UNDERSTANDING THYROID BLOOD WORK

- To evaluate the function of the thyroid gland, a full thyroid profile must be done.

- It should include:

- T4 and free T4 – reflect the availability of the storage form of the thyroid hormone

- T3 and free T3 – reflect the availability of the active form of the thyroid hormone

- Reverse T3 – is the inactive form of the thyroid hormone, which may block receptors (gates, which allow thyroid hormone to enter the cell where it will be used)

- There is another test commonly associated with the evaluation of thyroid function: TSH (thyroid-stimulating hormone). The TSH is not a product of the thyroid but is made by another gland in the body, the pituitary gland. TSH regulates the production of thyroid hormones. If the body needs more thyroid hormones, the pituitary gland produces more TSH. If there is too much thyroid hormone, TSH will go down. In general, the TSH level is inversely related to the function of the thyroid.

- Unfortunately, often, the only thyroid screening blood test done is the TSH.

TREATMENT OF THYROID DISEASE

- Hyperthyroidism (high thyroid function)

- Usually treated by an endocrinologist – a specialist who treats hormonal problems.

- Possible treatment options are treated with radioactive iodine, a surgery that removes the thyroid gland partially or totally, anti-thyroid medications (such as methimazole [Tapazole] and propylithiouracil). All those treatments work either through partial destruction of the excessive thyroid gland tissue or by suppressing the production of thyroid hormones.

- Beta-blockers – medications known as blood-pressure medications, which can be prescribed to control symptoms of hyperthyroidism, such as fast heart rate.

- Hypothyroidism (low thyroid function)

- Often treated by a primary care provider.

- Insufficient production of hormone managed with thyroid hormone supplementation. The most common drugs of choice are levothyroxine (Synthroid). Synthroid is a synthetic T4 hormone. It does not have any other thyroid hormones. For many people, Levothyroxine is a sufficient choice for therapy. However, regular blood work with a full thyroid profile is advised for monitoring the response to Synthroid.

TSH does not always reflect the functional status of the thyroid hormone's availability and should not be used as a single monitoring criterion.

CONVENTIONAL VS. FUNCTIONAL MEDICINE APPROACH TO HYPOTHYROIDISM MANAGEMENT

- Functional medicine practitioners believe FT3 is the most important indicator of optimal thyroid function and optimal thyroid hormone replacement. If there is enough of T4, but FT3 is low, the cells may still be suffering from insufficiency in thyroid hormones, and the patient may be symptomatic. Such a situation occurs because the conversion of T4 into T3 is altered. The possible cause of altered T4 to T3 conversion can be deficiency or insufficiency of iodine; zinc, selenium, copper; vitamin A; vitamins B2, B3, B6; vitamin C; vitamin D; and coenzyme Q10.

- Except for the vitamin D level, which is lately becoming part of the routine screening of most primary care providers, other factors as above are almost never checked by conventional providers and rarely associated with thyroid function work up. If your blood work indicates you have a poor T4 to T3 conversion, consider checking the levels of your vitamins or take supplements that support thyroid function.

- There is a Synthroid alternative that may be used. Armour Thyroid is a medication made from animal thyroid glands and was widely used before Synthroid dominated the market. Armour Thyroid and its compounding analogs contain the full spectrum of thyroid hormones and may be preferable for people who have poor T4 to T3 conversion. This medication is the preferred choice by functional medical providers.

REFERENCES

Barrett Barbie, Andrew Jurow, Kris Hart, Ron Rothenberg. 2019. Chap. 3 in Thyroid at Hormonal Bioidentity. (Barrowberg Press, 2019), 27–03.

Garber Jeffrey R., 1, 2, * Rhoda H. Cobin,3 Hossein Gharib,4 James V. Hennessey,2 Irwin Klein,5 Jeffrey I. Mechanick,6 Rachel Pessah-Pollack,6,7 Peter A. Singer, et al. "Clinical Practice Guidelines for Hypothyroidism in Adults: Cosponsored by the American Association of Clinical Endocrinologists and the American Thyroid Association." Thyroid 22, no. 12 (2012) [a] Mary Ann Liebert, Inc. doi:10.1089/thy.2012.0205.

Kawicka, Anna, and Bożena Regulska-llow. "Metabolic disorders and nutritional status in autoimmune thyroid diseases." Postepy Higieny i Medycyny Doswiadczlanej 69 (2015): 80–90. eISSN 1732-2693.

Ventura, Mara, 1 Miguel Melo,1,2 and Francisco Carrilho1Selenium and Thyroid Disease. Pathophysiology to Treatment International Journal of Endocrinology (2017): 9.

Yeung J. Meei, and Jonathan W. Serpell. "Management of the Solitary Thyroid Nodule." The Oncologist 13 (2008): 105–112.

EASY GUIDE TO SUGAR PROBLEMS

ALTHOUGH THE PHRASE, "SUGAR PROBLEMS," IS MOST USED IN REFERENCE TO DIABETES, THE PROBLEM IS MORE ADVANCED AND STARTS LONG BEFORE THE DIAGNOSTIC CRITERIA FOR DIABETES HAS BEEN MET. EARLY DETECTION OF THE CHANGES IN GLUCOSE METABOLISM IS VERY IMPORTANT BECAUSE, IN THE EARLY STAGE, THOSE CHANGES ARE COMPLETELY REVERSIBLE WITH DIET AND LIFESTYLE MODIFICATION.

THERE ARE THREE KNOWN TYPES OF DIABETES: TYPE 1, TYPE 2, AND GESTATIONAL DIABETES.

TO BE ABLE TO UNDERSTAND THE DIFFERENCES BETWEEN THOSE TYPES OF DIABETES, YOU NEED TO UNDERSTAND HOW THE HUMAN BODY USES SUGAR.

- Our body absorbs sugar in the form of glucose within the stomach and small intestine. Glucose is the primary fuel of our body. To be used, glucose needs to be moved into the cell. Glucose cannot enter the cell on its own but must be transported by insulin. The molecule of insulin signals the cell to open and let the glucose in by attaching it to insulin receptors. Think of the glucose molecule as a barge, an insulin molecule as a tow ship, and the receptor as a gate to the port. If any steps during this process fail, the glucose will continue to circulate in the blood and later transform into long-term storage. The cells will not receive "food" and will remain starved.

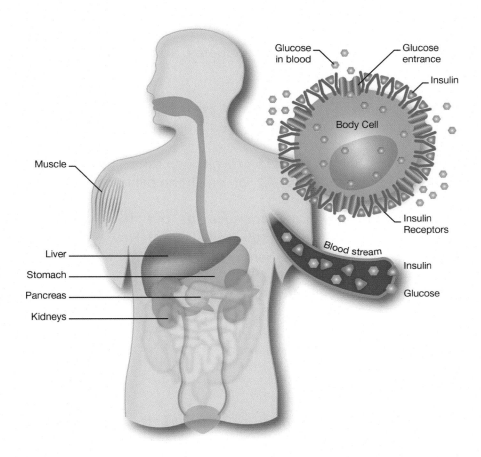

Glucose in blood

Glucose entrance

Insulin

Body Cell

Insulin Receptors

Muscle

Liver

Stomach

Pancreas

Kidneys

Blood stream

Insulin

Glucose

THERE ARE TWO MAJOR CAUSES OF BLOOD GLUCOSE DISEASE:

1. **THE BODY MAY NOT PRODUCE ENOUGH INSULIN DUE TO THE FAILURE OF THE PANCREATIC GLAND.**

2. **THE PROBLEM MAY OCCUR AT THE SITE OF THE INSULIN RECEPTOR, CAUSING INSULIN RESISTANCE (THE BARGE CANNOT ENTER THE PORT).**

- Type 1 diabetes is caused by the insufficient production of insulin in the pancreatic gland.

- Its onset is early in life, usually during childhood or adolescence.

- The only treatment for this type of diabetes are insulin injections and lifestyle modifications in the early stages.

- Although diet and a healthy lifestyle are advised and helpful, insulin is a critical component of the therapy and must be used lifelong.

- Gestational diabetes is an elevation of blood glucose, which develops during pregnancy. It is divided into class A1 and class A2, of which the pills do not control the sugar.

- Class A1 can be managed with diet and exercise, but class A2 usually needs insulin. Gestational diabetes is resolved after the baby is born. However, it is considered to be a strong risk factor for the development of DM type 2 in the future.

- Type 2 diabetes (DM) develops because of the failure to utilize insulin at the cellular level.

- Its onset is during midlife or the later years.

- Can be controlled with low-

- Will respond to anti-glycemic (lowering sugar) pills. Those medications are usually a choice during initial therapy.

- Insulin injections can be added to the treatment if the disease progressed to a certain stage.

Insulin also can be used for the short-term management of DM type 2 in special situations, such as during hospitalization for acute disease or during the management of the mother with a preexisting DM type 2 during the pregnancy.

THE MAIN SUBJECT OF THIS GUIDE IS THE CHANGES OF THE GLUCOSE METABOLISM ASSOCIATED WITH TYPE 2 DIABETES'S PATH. TYPE 2 DM IS THE MOST COMMON AMONG THIS DISEASE GROUP. THE PATHOLOGICAL MECHANISM OF DEVELOPING AND THE PROGRESSION OF TYPE 2 DM IS ALSO RESPONSIBLE FOR A NUMBER OF OTHER CHRONIC DISEASES.

- How does it happen?

- The diagnosis for diabetes is established based on laboratory tests. According to the American Diabetes Association, diagnostic criteria include the following:

- A fasting plasma glucose (FPG) level of 126 mg/dL (7.0 mmol/L) or higher, or

- a two-hour plasma glucose level of 200 mg/dL (11.1 mmol/L) or higher during a 75g oral glucose tolerance test (OGTT), or

- random plasma glucose of 200 mg/dL (11.1 mmol/L) or higher in a patient with the classic symptoms of hyperglycemia or hyperglycemic crisis, or

- a hemoglobin A1c (HbA1c) level of 6.5% (48 mmol/mol) or higher.

Changes in sugar metabolism start a long time before blood work reflects them. Usually, the body can compensate for glucose elevation for a while, and the measurable glucose elevation indicates the progression of the disease, not the disease beginning.

- Under the influence of certain internal and external factors, the normal levels of insulin produced by the pancreatic gland become unable to provide entry of the glucose into the cells normally. Blood glucose and insulin remain in the bloodstream, but the cells are still signaling the pancreatic gland to produce more insulin. This condition is called *insulin resistance*. The pancreatic gland responds to those signals and gives more insulin, causing *hyperinsulemia* (elevated amount of insulin). Excessive insulin leads to a drop in sugar in the blood (possible cause hypoglycemia, low-sugar state), which leads to the malfunctioning of the insulin receptors (the "gates" get broken and do not open any more), and over exhort the beta cells in the pancreas (those are the ones that produce insulin). If the situation repeats frequently, eventually, the pancreatic cells would burn out and would not be able to compensate for the abnormal demand for insulin. This would be the point when laboratory results start to show blood glucose elevation. Depending on the levels of those elevations, a diagnosis of *prediabetes* (Hg A1C 5.7–6.4) or diabetes (HgA1C > or = 6.5) is established.

RISK FACTORS ASSOCIATED WITH GLUCOSE METABOLISM DISEASE

- Genetic predisposition. Diabetes risk is hereditary. However, it may be significantly contained with proper diet and lifestyle modification.

- Chronic stress. Stress hormones interact with insulin. Chronic stress leads to alteration of insulin utilization.

- Altered sleep patterns. Insulin interacts with hormones regulating the sleep-and-activity cycle. Late-night bedtime, working at night, not enough sleep lead to alteration of insulin utilization.

- Excessive weight. The adipose tissue (fat) itself is involved in the endocrine activity. Obesity, especially abdominal obesity, is a strong risk factor for DM development. On the other hand, insulin resistance is a leading factor in fat metabolism alteration and in the progression of obesity itself.

- Dietary habits and choices are important. As earlier discussed, the progression of DM is stimulated by episodes of hyperglycemia provoked by eating high-carb meals (sweets, sweet fruits, bread, most traditional side dishes), causing a high demand for insulin overproduction that leads to developing more resistance.

- Alcohol is a "super sugar." Among other negative effects, overconsumption of alcohol predisposes one to develop problems with sugar.

- Insulin resistance changes the very process of breaking down glucose inside the cell (in the mitochondria). This biochemical process becomes less effective in energy production and produces more waste, causing the overproduction of oxygen-reactive species (ROS), inflammatory proteins, and states of chronic inflammation (not to be confused with infections), which can be seen in blood work as elevated ESR and CRP. Chronic inflammation became a hot topic in medical research over the last decade and now is linked to many chronic conditions. Two of the strongest and most dangerous links are the links to cardiovascular disease and neurodegenerative brain disease.

- Signs of blood sugar elevation (acute and chronic):

- Thirsty and dry mouth.

- Frequent urination, a full bladder sensation.

- Change of patterns in appetite.

- Hunger.

- Diminished energy levels.

- Shaking or sweating.

- Falling asleep after eating.

- Dizziness.

- Unexplained weight change. Weight loss is possible due to protein wasting. Weight gain is possible due to the development of excessive fat storage of underutilized glucose.

- Poor skin healing.

- Frequent infections, especially UTI.

- Vaginal yeast infections.

- Sexual dysfunction.

- Signs of low blood sugar (acute and chronic)

- Irritability, anxiety.

- Changes in the level of consciousness during acute low sugar episodes.

- Persistent fatigue.

- Episodes of unexplainable "not feeling well" 60–90 minutes after eating a high-carbohydrate food.

- Sugar craving

- Unexplained weight changes.

Blood glucose can be checked at home using a personal glucometer. For people with an established diagnosis of diabetes or prediabetes, a glucometer will be prescribed by most of the primary care providers. However, a glucometer can be bought in the pharmacy without a prescription if needed.

	Fasting	After eating	2-3 h after meal
Normal	80-100	170-200	120-140
Pre- Diabetic	101-125	190-230	140-160
Diabetic	126+	220-300	200+

Blood Glucose Chart

INSULIN RESISTANCE: DIET AND LIFESTYLE MODIFICATION

Those interventions are reasonable and appropriate for any stage of the type 2 glucose metabolism disease, including insulin resistance, prediabetes, and diabetes itself.

<u>Maintain a normal weight.</u> The medical criterion for normal weight is a BMI (body mass index) between 20 and 25. A lower BMI is often associated with wasting of the muscles. High BMI is associated with overweight and obesity. For obese individuals, losing at least 7 percent of body weight is linked to the improvement of HgA1C.

<u>Eat high-protein, low-carb food.</u> High-carb food is provocative to hyperinsulinemia state, and it leads to the progression of insulin resistance. Not all the food absorbed is the same. Carbohydrates absorb fast, and the changes in sugar levels in the blood are abrupt. High-protein food absorbs slowly. It does not cause hyperinsulinemia and helps to control symptoms associated with insulin resistance.

<u>Have sufficient amounts of healthy fats.</u> The poorly researched recommendation of a low-fat/high-carb diet had dominated Western society since the second half of the twentieth century. Several generations grow up with a false impression of fat being evil. The most recent research proved that healthy fats are needed for normal body functioning and are preventive against glucose metabolism problems. Fats provide alternative sources of energy, which involves different biochemical processes than glucose metabolism. Healthy fats are

cardioprotective, anti-inflammatory, and are needed for the utilization of fat-soluble vitamins and needed for healthy hormones.

Exercise. Physical activity of at least 150 min/week is an evidence-based recommendation for diabetes prevention.

Reduce stress, have sufficient sleep, and a normal circadian rhythm (sleeping-and-waking cycle). Stress, poor or insufficient sleep, and reversed circadian rhythms are interconnected to insulin resistance through the HPA axis (hypothalamic-pituitary-adrenal endocrine chain). Dysfunction of the HPA axis leads to weight gain, fatigue, abdominal obesity, cardio-metabolic disease, and neurodegeneration. It is important to have a healthy sleeping-and-waking cycle.

Testing for glucose metabolism disorders.

To access your blood glucose status, lab works are recommended. You will need to know:

Blood glucose level. This test reflects the level of blood glucose at the moment the blood is drawn. Limited conclusion.

HgA1C. This test reflects blood glucose levels as it's been over three months before the drawing of blood. If HgA1C is LOW, consider taking an INSULIN LEVEL test. Insulin levels have to check thirty minutes after a 75g glucose load for the earliest detection of glucose metabolism changes. Fasting insulin levels become elevated once the disease progresses. As it's been discussed earlier, the elevation of insulin levels is the first change measurable in the blood associated with dysmetabolic glucose disease. If the Hg A1C is high, a diagnosis of prediabetes or diabetes is established and appropriate treatment has to be initiated.

Thyroid hormone profile. Hypothyroidism (low function of the thyroid hormones) may lead to elevation of blood glucose (secondary diabetes).

Glucose in the urine. Excessive sugar is being eliminated through urination. The presence of glucose in the urine is a bad sign.

Those tests above are common, and most providers will do them routinely. There are several more tests that are not very common and are mostly considered by functional medicine providers.

<u>Saliva hormone testing</u> measures the sex hormones in the blood and cortisol at four points during one day. This test gives valuable information regarding your hormonal balance and the functioning of your hormone receptors (measuring hormones that had passed into the saliva gland as an opposite to the hormones circulating in the blood), and it measures the level of cortisol four times a day. Cortisol is the hormone that regulates the sleeping-and-waking cycle and stress response. It has a direct influence on insulin and glucose utilization.

<u>Zinc and chromium</u> are the trace elements directly linked to the normal function of insulin receptors as they transport glucose into the cell. The level of zinc and chromium is rarely checked in routine blood work.

<u>Vitamin D</u> deficiency is linked to glucose metabolic disease through the role of vitamin D in the normal function of beta cells in pancreatic gland

<u>Vitamins of group B: biotin (B7), thiamin (B1), cobalamin (B12)</u> have well-established evidence of insufficiency/deficiency in the diabetic population. Of those, only vitamin B12 is a common part of blood work.

<u>Adiponectin</u> is a protein that increases BEFORE insulin increases but drops low as the disease progresses.

Recommended blood work for insulin resistance evaluation: adiponectin, pro-insulin, HgA1C, fasting insulin, fasting blood glucose, CRP-HS, comprehensive metabolic profile, CBC. Additional testing: vitamin D, homocysteine, Apolipoprotein B, and Apolipoprotein A1.

Pharmacological treatment of glucose metabolism disorders

Medications for prediabetes and diabetes should be started if diet and lifestyle modifications are not enough to control blood glucose elevation.

The most common first-choice medication for prediabetes and type 2 diabetes is Metformin. The ADA 2020 guide to DM care recommends "Metformin therapy for prevention of type 2 diabetes should be considered in those with prediabetes, especially for those with BMI > =35 kg/m2, those aged, 60 years, and women with prior gestational diabetes mellitus." Metformin is one of the oldest sugar-control medications on market. It is also being discussed as a possible agent of anti-aging therapy. Metformin may affect kidney function and may decrease vitamin B12 levels. Proper monitoring with periodical blood work is recommended.

There are numerous choices of anti-glycemic medications on the market. Overall, it's important to understand about diabetic pills—they do not cure diabetes, but control sugar elevation. They need to be taken regularly, possibly lifelong. If blood sugar is controlled, it means the medication is doing a good job, but if the medication is stopped, blood glucose will go back to high levels. Elevated blood glucose does constant damage to the blood vessels, nerves, eyes, kidneys and leads to secondary diseases. Controlling elevated blood glucose levels is preventive to these complications.

INSULIN

Insulin therapy is a topic worthy of a book itself. There are several general principles about what is important in therapy.

Insulin administration MUST be coordinated to a mealtime. Insulins have ONSET (start working), PEAK (work most intensely), and DURATION (wear off). Depending on the type of insulin, this schedule may have significantly differed.

Types of Insulin

Insulin type	How it is delivered	Expiration when opened	Onset	Peak	Duration
Rapid Acting					
Admelog	Pens and vials	28 days	15-30 min	30 min-2 ½ hours	4-5 hours
Afrezza inhaled powder	4, 8 and 12 unit Cartridges	3 days	3-7 minutes	12-15 min	1 ½-3 hours
Apidra	Vials and pens	28 days	10-20 min	30 min-1 ½ hours	2-4 hours
Fiasp	Vials and pens	28 days	15-20 min	1 ½- 2 hours	5 hours
Humalog, U-100 and U-200	Vials, pens, cartridges for refillable pen	28 days	10-20 min	30 min-1/12 hours	3-5 hours
Novolog	Vials, pens, cartridges for refillable pen	28 days	10-20 min	1-3 hours	3-5 hours
Short Acting **	Vials and pens				
Regular		31-42 days, depending upon brand	15-30 min	2 ½-5 hours	4-12 hours
U-500 (5x the concentration)	Vials and pens	28 days	30 min	4-8 hours	18-24 hours
Intermediate acting **	Vials and pens				
NPH (created in 1946)		31-42 days, depending upon brand	1-2 hours	4-12 hours	14-24 hours
Long acting					
Basaglar	Vials and pens	28 days	3-4 hours	No peak +	11-24 hours
Lantus	Vials and pens	28 days	3-4 hours	No peak +	11-24 hours
Levemir	Vials and pens	42 days	3-4 hours	No peak +	6-23 hours
Toujeo, U-300	Pen only	42 days	6 hours	No peak	24-36 hours
Tresiba, U-100 and U-200	Pen only	56 days	1 hour	9 hours	36-42 hours
Combination					
NPH/Regular 70/30	Vials and pens	31-42 d vial 10 d pen	30 min	50 min-2 hours and 6-10 hours	18-24 hours
Rapid acting 70/30	Vials and pens	28 d vial 14 d pen	15-30 min	1-4 hours	18-24 hours
Rapid acting 75/25	Vials and pens	28 d vial 10 d pen	15-30 min	1-6 ½ hours	12-24 hours
Rapid acting 50/50	Vials and pens	28 d vial 10 d pen	15-30 min		

As it is easy to see from the table, it is important to know how YOUR insulin works and to have meals within the period of insulin activity.

Understanding the differences between insulins are also useful if you need injections more than once a day. Choosing insulin to pick during the hours of your most demand for insulin may help to improve glucose control and minimize periods of uncontrolled hyperglycemia (high sugar) and hypoglycemia (low sugar). Your goal is to be within the normal range of blood glucose around the clock.

SUPPLEMENTS SUPPORTING GLUCOSE UTILIZATION

- Berberine, a naturally occurring alkaloid found in a number of plants, is an effective supplement for helping to maintain cardio-metabolic health.

- Alpha-lipoic acid (ALA) – Doses of 600 to 1800mg/day can improve insulin sensitivity; doses 600–1200mg improve circulation and diabetic polyneuropathy.

- Trace elements supplementation has several benefits. Chromium (dose of 1000mcg/day) and zinc benefit normal the function of insulin receptors and glucose transport.

- Vitamin D (doses between 2000 and 5000IU a day) is appropriate. Blood test monitoring is advised to individual therapeutic dose established.

- Magnesium (200–400mg/day) needs if insufficiency/deficiency present. Blood work can help evaluate levels of magnesium in the blood.

- Coenzyme Q10 has an important role in cardiac health, insulin resistance control, thyroid hormone function optimization, and mitochondria function. The recommended dose calculation is 100mg if you are age >50; 100+mg when high blood pressure, cardiac disease, high cholesterol, or diabetes is present; 100+mg if you have more than one of these diseases; 100+mg if you take cholesterol medications or blood pressure medications. The dose is between 100 and 400mg a day.

REFERENCES

Vagnini, Frederic J., and Mary Infantino. Diabetes: Facts, Diagnosis, and treatment. Guide to Anti-Aging &Regenerative Medicine 2013–2018. Chap. 17. (American Academy of Anti-Aging Medicine), 471–498.

Trindade, Filomena. The Continuum of Insulin Resistance: Guide to Anti-Aging & Regenerative Medicine 2013–2018. Chapter 18. (American Academy of Anti-Aging Medicine), 499–544.

Anastasopoulou, Catherine, ed. "Type 2 Diabetes Diagnostic Criteria" Buck Christensen ADA, https://emedicine.medscape.com/article/2172154-overview

Standard of Medical Care Diabetes—2020 www.diabetes.org/diabetescare

Abbott, Sabra M., and Roneil G. Malkani, Phyllis C. Zee. "Circadian disruption and human health: A bidirectional relationship." European Journal of Neuroscience 51, no. 1 (2020): 567–583. doi:10.1111/ejn. 14298.

Moreno, Claudia R.C.1, 2*, Elaine C. MARQUEZE3, Charli SARGENT4, Kenneth P. WRIGHT Jr5, Sally A. Ferguson,4 and Philip Tucker2, 6 "Working Time Society consensus statements: Evidence-based effects of shift work on physical and mental health." Industrial Health 57 (2019): 139–157.

Anderson, R A. "Nutritional factors influencing the glucose/insulin system: chromium." Journal of the American College of Nutrition 16, no. 5 (1997).

Via, Michael. "The Malnutrition of Obesity: Micronutrient Deficiencies That Promote Diabetes." Endocrinology (2012): 8. doi:10.5402/2012/103472

EASY GUIDE TO UNDERSTANDING WEIGHT LOSS

WEIGHT LOSS, WHAT IS IT?

Weight loss is an exciting topic for many people. But before we move to the practical aspect of weight loss, let's understand the very definition of what we mean by weight loss.

Oxford Dictionary defines weight loss as a "decrease in body weight."

There are several possible causes for weight loss: dehydration, loss of muscular mass, or loss of fat mass.

It is important to understand that the goal of medical weight loss is to benefit your future health. And medical weight loss means losing excessive fat mass and changing your body composition to reduce fat and increase lean mass.

Weight loss is always a systemic process, and fat will be reduced all over the body.

It is not uncommon that a person has a localized fat deposit, which esthetically disagrees with his/her self-image. If this person is within normal weight and attempts weight loss intervention to correct a localized problem, the results will be disappointing. There are other ways to take care of local fat, generally called **body countering**.

Body contouring methods include surgical liposuction, fat freezing (such as coolsculpting), fat-burning (SculpSure is an example), or chemical burning of the fat (such as kybella). All these methods lead to the correction of a cosmetic defect but do not improve overall body weight and, as such, has no future health benefits.

It is important to understand the benefits of both methods and use them correctly.

IDEAL BODY WEIGHT AND BODY COMPOSITION: UNDERSTAND YOUR CURRENT SITUATION. BELOW ARE REFERENCE CHARTS FOR YOU TO DETERMINE YOUR IDEAL BODY WEIGHT, BODY COMPOSITION, AND BODY MASS INDEX (BMI) CLASSIFICATION.

- Estimate Ideal body weight in (kg)

    Males: IBW = 50 kg + 2.3 kg for each inch over 5 feet.

    Females: IBW = 45.5 kg + 2.3 kg for each inch over 5 feet.

    (https://globalrph.com/medcalcs/adjusted- body-weight-ajbw-and-ideal-body-weight-ibw-calc/)

ACE Body Fat Percent Norms for Men and Women

Description	Women	Men
Essential Fat	10% to 13%	2% to 5%
Athletes	14% to 20%	6% to 13%
Fitness	21% to 24%	14% to 17%
Acceptable	25% to 31%	18% to 24%
Obese	Over 32%	Over 25%

Healthy Body Composition
The American Council on Exercise (ACE) gives the following ranges of values for different populations.

- Body mass index (BMI) is a person's weight in kilograms divided by the square of their height in meters. A high BMI can be an indicator of high body fatness.

- If your BMI is less than 18.5, it falls within the underweight range.

- If your BMI is 18.5 to <25, it falls within the normal.

- If your BMI is 25.0 to <30, it falls within the overweight range.

- If your BMI is 30.0 or higher, it falls within the obese range.

- Obesity is frequently subdivided into categories:

- Class 1: BMI of 30 to < 35

- Class 2: BMI of 35 to < 40

- Class 3: BMI of 40 or higher. Class 3 obesity is sometimes categorized as "extreme" or "severe" obesity.

https://www.cdc.gov/obesity/adult/defining.html

SETTING YOUR WEIGHT LOSS GOAL USING BODY COMPOSITION MEASUREMENT

THE HEALTHY WEIGHT GOAL IS TO BE WITHIN YOUR NORMAL WEIGHT RANGE

- Cosmetic weight loss leads to yo-yo dieting, regaining weight to an increase of excessive weight, worsening the general health and causing emotional disappointment.

- There are two examples of body composition analyses and the interpretation of those findings.

```
         TANITA
    BODY COMPOSITION
        ANALYZER
         TBF-410
BODY TYPE        STANDARD
GENDER             FEMALE
AGE                    50
HEIGHT           5ft 3.0in
WEIGHT             168.0lb
BMI                  29.8
BMR              6061   kJ
                 1449kcal
IMPEDANCE         532   Ω
FAT%               41.0%
FAT MASS           68.8lb
FFM                99.2lb
TBW                72.6lb
DESIRABLE RANGE
FAT%               23-34%
FAT MASS       29.6-51.2lb
```

```
         TANITA
    BODY COMPOSITION
        ANALYZER
         TBF-410
BODY TYPE        STANDARD
GENDER             FEMALE
AGE                    41
HEIGHT           5ft 2.0in
WEIGHT             108.8lb
BMI                  19.9
BMR              5139   kJ
                 1228kcal
IMPEDANCE         734   Ω
FAT%               25.9%
FAT MASS           28.2lb
FFM                80.6lb
TBW                59.0lb
DESIRABLE RANGE
FAT%               23-34%
FAT MASS       24.0-41.6lb
```

Person #1: BMI 29.8 overweight

Fat mass 68.8, must be between 29.6 and 51.21. 68.8 lb.–51.21lb. =17.6 lb. – minimal fat loss goal.

Optimal fat mass must be in the middle of the normal fat range:

10+ lb. – It's bringing a weight loss goal of 27.6 lb. of fat. Ten percent of weight loss will come from nonfat tissue: 3+ lb. Weight loss goal: 31 lb.

Person #2: BMI 19.9. Underweight. Not a candidate for weight loss.

WHY THE DIET IS A MUST?

FAT LOSS WILL NOT OCCUR

UNLESS YOUR BODY HAS NEEDS TO USE THE STORED FAT FOR ENERGY. WHAT IT MEANS IS THAT A PERSON WHO WANTS TO LOSE WEIGHT NEEDS TO CONSUME FEWER CALORIES THAN THE AMOUNT THAT IS SPENT TO SUSTAIN LIFE AND ACTIVITIES.

"Lipolysis is the metabolic mechanism our body uses to break down lipids into fatty acid. Our body employs this mechanism than it needs to use stored fat for energy production."

"One pound of fat is equal to approximately 3,500 cal. To lose one pound of fat, a person needs to spend approximately 3,500 calories."

Your weight loss rate will depend on how fast you can achieve this deficit.

It is highly unlikely anyone can achieve it in one day because, for most people, the calories daily need is less than 3,500. However, if you will underwrite 500 calories every day, you will achieve the deficit of 3,500 calls within 7 days.

It is recommended to combine dieting and exercise as your tools for healthy weight loss.

MANY POPULAR DIETS HAVE GOALS OTHER THEN WEIGHT LOSS. THEY STILL CAN BE USED FOR WEIGHT LOSS IN COMBINATION WITH CALORIE RESTRICTION.

PALEOLITHIC DIET HAS THE ADVANTAGE OF OTHER DIETS: PLEASURE TO EAT, NO JUNK FOOD SINCE JUNK FOOD IS PROCESSED FOOD, GOOD RANGE OF FOOD CHOICES, A LOT OF VEGETABLES, LOW IN TOXIC FATS, NO EXCESSIVE CARBS, PERIODS OF FASTING, FOODS SEPARATION.

THE DIET'S PRIMARY GOAL IS GOOD NUTRITION AND HEALTHY BODY.

- Low-fat diets are diets that dramatically limit the grams of fat a person is allowed to consume throughout the day. Low-fat diets, though useful for short-term weight loss, may not be healthy or successful in the long-term. The benefits of a low-fat diet are much contested and many studies have found very little, if any benefit. For example, an eight-year trial of almost 49,000 women, called the Women's Health Initiative (WHI) Dietary Modification Trial, found that a low-fat diet had no effect on breast cancer, heart disease, colorectal cancer, or weight. A study published in the October 2015 issue of the journal, The Lancet Diabetes & Endocrinology, found that low-fat diets are also of no use for long-term weight loss.

THE PROLON FASTING MIMICKING DIET IS THE FIRST AND ONLY MEAL PROGRAM THAT HAS GONE THROUGH CLINICAL TRIALS AT THE UNIVERSITY OF SOUTHERN CALIFORNIA AND HAS BEEN PATENTED FOR ITS <u>ANTI- AGING EFFECTS</u>! THIS 5-DAY MEAL PROGRAM PROVIDES SCIENTIFICALLY RESEARCHED MICRO- AND MACRO-NUTRIENTS IN PRECISE QUANTITIES AND COMBINATIONS THAT NOURISH YOU BUT ARE NOT RECOGNIZED AS FOOD BY YOUR BODY AND, THEREFORE, MIMICS A FASTING STATE!

<u>HTTPS://PROLONFMD.COM/FASTING-MIMICKING-DIET</u>

- Intermittent fasting is an eating pattern where you cycle between periods of eating and fasting. It does not say anything about which foods to eat, but rather when you should eat. You're technically fasting for sixteen hours every day and restricting your eating to an eight-hour eating window. This is the most popular form of intermittent fasting, known as the 16/8 method. No food is allowed during the fasting period, but you can drink water, coffee, tea, **and other non-**

- This diet has the primary goal of restoring normal cell function, mitochondria and receptors recovery.

CALORIE RESTRICTION: IS THIS THE ONLY FACTOR? NO

Key Disturbances that Contribute to Fat Gain

- Gut/immune balance

- Chronic inflammation

- Nutrient deficiencies

- Infections –including mold, biotoxins

- Carb and sugar intake (glucose balance)

- Cortisol – stress

- Cortisol – sleep

- Craving – reward – satiety Low metabolic performance (thyroid) intoxication / Kidneys-Liver-Lymph Sex hormones

- Drug use

- Social and community cues

(From a lecture by James LaValle RPH, CCN, MT, ND "Metabolism of Weight Loss and Fasting.")

Medications which may affect gut microbiome:

Antibiotics

NSAIDs (over-the-counter painkillers)

Corticosteroids (often are being prescribed for asthma therapy)

Ox/HRT (birth control pills)

PPI/H2 blockers (heartburn and stomach medications)

Metformin

Stations (cholesterol medications)

Antipsychotic

Opioids

Lab test recommended for proper evaluation of obesity and weight loss

- Waking serum cortisol or 4-point salivary

- DHEAs

- Siege thyroid profile T4, T3 free and total, TSH, TPO Thyroglobulin AB Blood glucose fasting, and glucometer 1-hour post-meal readings

- RBC magnesium

- RBC chromium

- Monocytes and Eosinophil%

- Triglycerides

EFFECTIVE WEIGHT LOSS IS MORE THAN CALORIES IN, CALORIES OUT

- Chronic inflammation is a long-term body state of inflammation, lasting from several months to years.

- It's not the same as an infection. May be provoked by some chronic infection. It manifests by losing the homeostatic balance of pro- and anti-inflammatory reactions at the cellular level, leading to the malfunction of the cell itself, the ineffective utilization of energy, and increased production of waste and toxicity. Can be detected with blood work. Excessive white fat tissue up-regulates the production of cytokines (large group of proteins, peptides, or glycoproteins that are secreted by specific cells of the immune system) and can become a reason for chronic inflammation on its own.

- Excessive fat tissue suppresses the growth hormone. Growth hormone is responsible for growing children. It continues to be produced in adulthood. For adults, it really becomes a hormone of recovery. It is important for many functions, including lean muscle mass development. Lean muscles are the biggest endocrine organ that utilizes glucose in large amounts and may reverse insulin resistance even for people who already have diabetes.

- Endocrine activity of the adipose (fat) tissue changes the mechanism of how we process glucose to less effect. As a result, energy production drops up to 90 percent, and toxin production increases. It leads to an increase in appetite, increase in inflammation, rise in blood pressure, change in lipid metabolism, decrease in insulin sensitivity.

EFFECTIVE WEIGHT LOSS IS MORE THAN CALORIES IN, CALORIES OUT

For the successful use of insulin, thyroid hormone, serotonin, and many other things in our body, we need specific cell receptors (the gates in the plasma membrane that opens up only to the substance it is designated for) functioning well. If the receptors are malfunctioning, we are facing a state of resistance (insulin resistance, serotonin resistance, T3 resistance, etc.)

At the state of resistance, our body cannot effectively utilize the named substance u if it has enough. Increasing the availability of the substance will not resolve the problem since the body still cannot use it. The higher concentration even may lead to higher resistance since the receptors will be "overwhelmed" and will "shut down" all the more.

There are many nutritional factors that may lead to receptors malfunctioning. The group of trace elements plays multiple roles in intracellular transport and conversion. The other important mineral is magnesium. A typical American diet often is deficient in magnesium.

For the intestinal absorption of nutrients and minerals influenced by healthy flora in the gut, probiotics may help to improve intestinal absorption and to correct nutritional imbalances.

Reward cascade: Low serotonergic and dopaminergic action is driving craving behaviors (increase craving and addiction). Obese individuals have low serum tryptophan. Tryptophan is a precursor of serotonin. Serotonin is important in calming and craving satisfaction. A low level of serotonin leads to cravings and unhappiness, which causes comfort and chain eating.

CHOOSING YOUR DIET

- Consider doing genetic testing. It may give you a good clue about which diet is right for you.

- Consider your daily routine patterns. Poor sleep influences levels and the interactions of your hormones. You need a good balance between work and rest time.

- Understand that your effective diet plan will most likely be long term. Choose a plan that allows you to eat food you enjoy.

- Consider doing lab work, evaluating your gut health.

- Consider lab work evaluation levels of your hormones, insulin, and long-term blood glucose.

- Consider taking supplements that contain trace elements.

Alcohol Metabolism
You are more likely to metabolize alcohol normally

Caffeine Metabolism
You are a slow caffeine metabolizer

Gluten Sensitivity
You are more likely to have gluten sensitivity

Lactose Intolerance
You have an increased likelihood of being lactose intolerant

Weight Management
You are more likely to become overweight

Carbohydrate Metabolism
You are more likely to be a slow carbohydrate metabolizer

Stress Eating
You are less prone to stress eating and snacking

Fat Metabolism and Body Weight
A low fat diet will not significantly help with your weight management efforts

Omega 3 Fatty Acids Levels
You have an increased likelihood of having lower omega-3 fatty acid levels

Triglyceride Levels
You have a moderate likelihood of elevated triglycerides

Weight Regain After Diet
You may be more prone to regain weight after dieting

Salt Sensitivity
A low sodium diet may significantly lower your blood pressure

Monounsaturated Fatty Acids Levels
You do not have an increased likelihood of low monounsaturated fatty acid levels

Cholesterol Levels
You have a moderate likelihood of elevated cholesterol

Saturated Fatty Acid Levels
You have an increased likelihood of elevated saturated fat levels

Polyunsaturated Fatty Acids Levels
You do not have an increased likelihood of having lower polyunsaturated fatty acid levels

DECISION MAKING: SOMETIMES YOU NEED MORE THAN DIET AND EXERCISE

- If your BMI is under 35, your chances for weight loss success through a diet and exercise program is very good.

- Between BMI 35 and 40, weight loss becomes more difficult, especially in the presence of other chronic diseases.

- Above 40, more aggressive methods may be a good option.

- Everyone must try active weight loss with diet, exercise, and possible supportive medical therapies for at least 6 months. If after 6 months you see no significant progress and your BMI >35, consider bariatric surgical consultation.

- Understand: Obesity is a progressive disease. If you see the progression of weight gain of at least 5 lb. a year over the last five years, this tendency is likely to continue in the future and will lead to the more advanced stage of obesity and to developing secondary health problems associated with obesity.

MEDICATION AND SUPPLEMENTS FOR WEIGHT LOSS SUPPORT

OTC (over-the-counter) weight loss supplement (nutritional supplements): Is NOT FDA approved for weight loss unless considered to be MEDICATION. **Alli** is the ONLY MEDICATION available OTC currently.

NUTRITIONAL SUPPLEMENTS can be divided into two groups: those promoting water loss and stimulants (any supplement that states, "Raising calorie and fat metabolism," is likely to be in this group). The first category does not really cause fat loss, only short-term water reduction. The second category has potential side effects of raising blood pressure and increasing heart rate. Those could be dangerous for people with existing cardiovascular disease or are predisposed to developing those conditions. Always read the label for active ingredients in the supplements.

All prescribed medication can be started only if a patient's BMI > 27.5. Even prescribed medications must be used as junction therapy with a diet and exercise program in place.

Phentermine (common brands Lomaira, Adipex-P): It can promote weight loss when used for a short time. Controlled substance. Can cause a rapid or irregular heartbeat, delirium, panic, psychosis, and heart failure. (https://drugfree.org/drug/prescription-stimulants/?utm_source=google&utm_medium=kp&utm_campaign=stimulants)

Belviq (lorcaserin) and **Contrave** (naltrexone HCl/bupropion HCl): treat obesity as food dependency. Most helpful for people with obsessive eating behaviors. Serious side effects of Contrave include risks of seizures. Both medications have the potential for aggravating mental health disorders and may interact with mental health medication. (https://www.belviq.com/en

(https://contrave.com/?gclid=Cj0KCQiAI5zwBRCTARIsAlrukdPxsQQ8ak4BOWH0INem RzHbU5MUuAGyiOedELQ H45XaCkZtJfDdAXMaAnt8EALw_wcB)

FUNCTIONAL MEDICINE WEIGHT LOSS SUPPLEMENT RECOMMENDATIONS

- Chromium: needed for normal function of insulin receptors.

- Magnesium: critical for 400 biochemical reactions. Low levels associated with insulin resistance and increased risk of prediabetes. If having problems with sleep, take at night.

- Vitamin D3: low vitamin D levels (17ng/ml and less), independent of all other risk factors, increased risk of death more than any other risk factored at 20.6% (Melamed ML, Michos ED, Post W, Astor B. "25-Hydroxyvitamin D levels and the Risk of Mortality in the General

Population." *Archives of Internal Medicine* 168 (2008):1629–1637). May help to upregulate insulin resistance, play a role in immune response, have an anti-neuro-inflammatory function, and play a role in the utilization of calcium and bone health.

Trace elements: plays a role in the healthy function of receptors, hormone conversion, immune response, and more.

Probiotics: to restore healthy gut flora, detoxification, improve nutrients absorption, and the correction of secondary problems associated with malabsorption and malnutrition.

- Adiponectin: improves glucose sensitivity, inhibits inflammatory cytokines, decreases the risk of a heart attack.

- Capsinoids: enhances white belly fat lipolysis, improves energy expenditure and metabolism, improves lipids oxygenation, may suppress appetite.

- Melatonin: improves sleep. Helps to restore cortisol balance.

- Evade: improves insulin sensitivity. Inhibits adipogenesis.

- White beans extract: clinically proven weight loss and body fat reduction. May reduce the enzymatic digestion of dietary starches.

- *Magnolia officinalis* and *Phellodendron amurense*: stress-related appetite control and fat deposition reduction; antianxiety; helps to normalize cortisol and DHEA levels, including induced by exercise; decreases food craving.

- ALA: improves insulin resistance, reduces the incidence/symptoms of neuropathy, improves heavy metal detoxification.

COMPOUNDING WEIGHT LOSS SUPPLEMENT

- Compounding products are made in compounding pharmacies and not available without prescriptions; those combinations had not been evaluated for effectiveness through official FDA investigation. However, it is backed up by scientific and medical research and has an established record of use in the medical practice.

- MIC (lipotropic injections): NOT causing weight loss but helps more effective weight loss process in diet/exercise-induced calorie-deficit condition. Three components always present at MIC injections:

- **Methionine**: it supports the digestive system by helping to remove heavy metals within the body while breaking down fat deposits. This prevents the possible buildup of fat in the arteries. Methionine also supports liver detoxification.

- **Inositol**: supports the transport of nutrients at the cellular level and helps maintain proper electrical energy across the cell membrane. Inositol converts fats into other useful forms of energy and assists in establishing healthy cell membranes, facilitating nerve impulses.

- **Choline**: assists in controlling cholesterol levels in the blood and controlling weight gain by maintaining healthy cell membranes. Choline has been linked to and directly associated with the maintenance of the nervous system, assisting memory, and is critical for normal cell membrane structure and function.

Other common ingredients within MIC injections are B vitamins and L-carnitine, which allows for

CONCLUSION

- There are more options for weight loss that were not covered in this guide. There are many choices, and there is the right choice for everyone.

- The most important thought the author of this guide wishes to bring to the reader is understanding that obesity is not just an aesthetic issue, it is a health issue. Untreated, this chronic illness WILL PROGRESS and WILL LEAD to diabetes, hypertension, musculoskeletal disease, and more. Even worse, it leads to social isolation, low self-esteem, and dissatisfaction in life. Everyone deserves a healthy and happy life. Take care of yourself. NO ONE but YOU can do it. We, health care workers, are here to help when you need us. The choice is yours. Be well.

EASY GUIDE TO UNDERSTANDING YOUR BODY AFTER BARIATRIC SURGERY: WHAT DO YOU NEED TO KNOW

ALL BARIATRIC SURGERIES CHANGE YOUR BODY FOREVER. THE BENEFITS OF THESE PROCEDURES ARE VERY CLEAR AND IN MANY CASES WEIGHT LOSS IS CRITICALLY IMPORTANT FOR FUTURE HEALTH PRESERVATION. AT THE SAME TIME, PEOPLE, AFTER THOSE PROCEDURES, HAVE SPECIAL NEEDS. IT IS IMPORTANT FOR BOTH THE PATIENT AND HIS/HER HEALTH CARE PROVIDER UNDERSTAND THOSE NEEDS AND ADDRESS THEM IN A TIMELY FASHION.

- All bariatric surgeries are divided into two categories: restrictive and restrictive.

- Restrictive surgeries reduce the size of the stomach. Lap band and gastric sleeve are restrictive surgeries.

- Restrictive-malabsorptive surgeries reduce the size of the stomach and limit the amount of nutrients the body absorbs by bypassing a portion of the

- small intestine. Gastric bypass and the duodenal switch are restrictive-malabsorption surgeries.

- The malabsorption at the second type of the surgeries is not a complication but an expected outcome. It plays a role in greater weight loss and the future maintenance of a healthy weight.

Adjustable Gastric Band
(Lap Band)

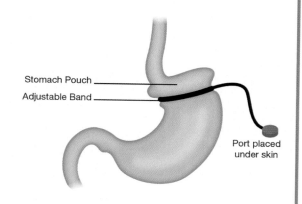

Stomach Pouch

Adjustable Band

Port placed
under skin

Roux-en-Y Gastric Bypass
(RNY)

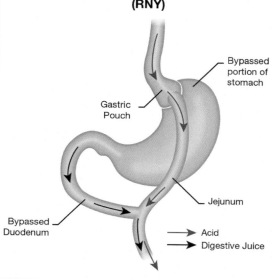

Bypassed
portion of
stomach

Gastric
Pouch

Jejunum

Bypassed
Duodenum

→ Acid
→ Digestive Juice

Duodenal Switch (DS)

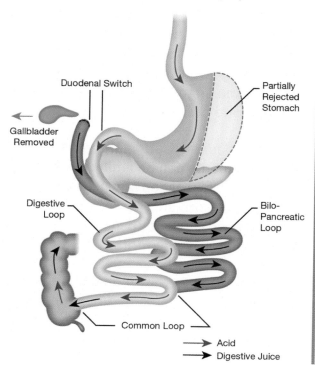

Duodenal Switch

Gallbladder
Removed

Partially
Rejected
Stomach

Digestive
Loop

Bilo-
Pancreatic
Loop

Common Loop

→ Acid
→ Digestive Juice

Vertical Sleeve Gastrectomy
(Gastric Sleeve)

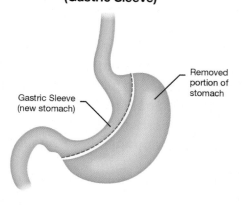

Gastric Sleeve
(new stomach)

Removed
portion of
stomach

SPECIAL NEEDS OF BARIATRIC SURGICAL SURVIVALS

- Malabsorption is common in all types of bariatric surgeries. Although restrictive-only surgeries are less likely to develop significant nutritional deficiencies, there are factors like reduced calorie intake, avoidance of nutrient-rich foods, persistent vomiting, and use of medications that reduce the ability to absorb nutrients. There is evidence that bariatric surgery changes the composition of intestinal microbes (friendly bacteria and funguses that normally live in our intestines and play an important role in the breakdown and absorption of the nutrients and even synthesize some vitamins for us). Dysbacteriosis is a factor that may lead to nutritional insufficiencies and deficiencies.

- Oral supplementation of vitamins and minerals is advised after all types of bariatric surgeries. However, the effectiveness of oral supplements can be limited by such factors as intolerance to pills (supplements often cause stomach irritation and nausea), the limited ability of the altered stomach and small intestine to absorb supplements (if the stomach cannot absorb those nutrients from the food, it will have similar difficulties to absorb them from supplements), poor quality of the supplements itself, and more.

- If oral supplementation is not enough, the other options for nutritional support may be considered, such as sublingual drops, nasal sprays, and creams and patches especially formulated for the nutritional support (do not confuse this option with skin care products). The most effective alternative to pills is injections and vitamins/mineral-mix intravenous infusions.

WHAT DEFICITS ARE MOST COMMON AND HOW THEY CAN AFFECT YOU

- There is a good research database that describes the most common deficiencies found after bariatric surgeries.

- The most common deficiency after bariatric surgery is a **<u>protein deficiency</u>**. Sufficient protein intake is considered a protection against the loss of lean body mass in any situation when rapid weight loss occurs. After bariatric surgery, protein absorption decreases because malabsorption delays the mix of the food with bile and digestive enzymes, low consumption, high-protein food, low amount of stomach acid. Hair loss, muscular weakness, and generalized fatigue are caused by this deficiency. Protein deficiency can be found during blood work. Blood works will show decreased *albumin, prealbumin, and total serum albumin*. To maintain healthy muscles, at least 30g of protein should be consumed in more than one meal.

- Malabsorption of the **<u>vitamin B12</u>** after bariatric surgery results in the decreased production of the stomach acid and reduced availability of *intrinsic factor*. Because the body usually stores Vitamin B12, this deficiency may not be seen immediately after the surgery but has a chance to develop in the second half of the first postsurgical year. This deficiency may be responsible for such symptoms as anemia (can be found in the blood work as low Hg and HCT), fatigue, changes in mental status, vision changes due to the damage in the optic nerve, and memory loss. Low Vitamin B12 may lead to secondary damage through the elevation of *homocysteine* (the fat in the blood considered to be an independent predictor of heart disease. If *homocysteine* is elevated, the person is at higher risk of heart attack and other complications of cardiovascular disease). Vitamin B12 levels are checked during blood work. Vitamin B12 is best replaced through injections or as a part of an IV vitamin infusion. The second best way to replace it is a nasal spray Nascobal. Vitamins B12 tablets have greater chances not to be absorbed well.

- **<u>Iron deficiency</u>** is a common finding after bariatric surgery. The risk even higher for women of childbearing age because of the blood loss associated with menstruation. The symptoms caused by conditions are anemia, fatigue, cracks in the corner of the mouth, difficulty in swallowing, swelling of the tongue, brittle nails, shortness of breath, and heart palpitation. Blood work indicating iron deficiency shows decreased *iron and ferritin*. Oral supplementation of iron can be challenging because this medication is well known for irritating the stomach even for people who do not have preexisting gastric problems. For a compromised postsurgical stomach, the side effect may become severe. If this is a case, IV iron infusion should be considered. Iron absorption is improved by a co-administration of vitamin C. Iron has to be taken on an empty stomach and milk products should be avoided for two hours before and after iron has been taking.

WHAT DEFICIENCIES ARE MOST COMMON AND HOW CAN THEY AFFECT YOU

- The risk **of thiamin (vitamin B1)** deficiency is increased in those patients who vomit a lot. This deficiency is dangerous and may lead to the fast development of neurological complications. **Wernicke encephalopathy** is an acute neurological condition characterized by a clinical triad of ophthalmoparesis with nystagmus (abnormal movement of the eyes), ataxia (muscle weakness and difficulty to control movement), and confusion. This is a life-threatening illness that needs to be treated in the hospital with IV thiamin protocol. **Korsakoff syndrome** is a chronic memory disorder, also caused by a vitamin B1 deficiency. Symptoms of vitamin B1 deficiency are muscular weakness, loss of reflexes, disturbance in coordination, pain in the extremities. The levels of *vitamin B1* can be checked during blood work. The warning part, this vitamin is almost never included in routine blood works by an average provider and often is being forgotten in the blood work of a post-bariatric patient if those blood orders are done by a provider who does not often care for post-bariatric patients. Take oral supplementation of this vitamin without food, avoid tea and coffee.

- **Folic acid (vitamin B9)** is yet another common deficiency for those post-bariatric with status. It also manifests as anemia, inflammation of the tongue, and tiredness. Blood work associated with this deficiency are *low folate, increase MCV, increase RDW, decreased RBC, and increase homocysteine*. Oral supplementation of folic acid usually works well. This vitamin is sensitive to alcohol, so alcohol needs to be avoided.

- **Vitamin C (ascorbic acid)** is poorly presented in the literature research of post-bariatric vitamin deficiency. However, the author of this guide saw mullet clinical cases of vitamin C deficiency associated with hair loss that is experienced by patients after bariatric surgery. Vitamin C is rarely checked in routine blood work, and for most laboratories, the specimen drawn requires a special vial and handling. If you want this vitamin level to be checked, you will have to request it from your health provider. Aside from hair preservation, vitamin C is important for immune supports and is a powerful antioxidant, which means anti-aging and skin maintenance benefits.

WHAT DEFICIENCIES ARE MOST COMMON AND HOW CAN THEY AFFECT YOU

- Absorption of **fat-soluble vitamins (vitamins A, E, K, D)** is reduced after bariatric surgery and leads to poor absorption of fat.

Among this group, vitamin D is one often discussed in the media and often prescribed by general practice health providers. The other vitamins in the fat-soluble group frequently overlook. Important to know, these vitamins depending on each other's support and cannot be fully utilized in the body if one of them is missing. As an example, to work the best to support calcium in the bones, vitamin D needs sufficient vitamin K. Otherwise, calcium will remain in the bloodstream, increasing the risk of calcification of the blood vessels. The receptors (gates into the cells) specifically for vitamin D depend on vitamin A. If you are taking a vitamin D supplement, but the levels of vitamin D remain low, consider checking vitamin A.

- Symptoms associated with those vitamins deficiencies are

- **vitamin D** ¬ bone pain, muscular weakness, difficulty in getting up from a chair of flat surface;

- **Vitamin A** – night blindness and vision change, dry skin, conjunctive dryness and keratin deposits on the conjunctiva, poor wound healing;

- **Vitamin K** – easy bleeding; and

- **Vitamin E** – anemia, changes in eye movements, tingling, numbness, and strange sensation in the distant extremities.

- For the exception of vitamin D, the other fat-soluble vitamins are rarely included in the routine blood work and will often still be forgotten to be included in the blood work for post-bariatric patients.

- Fat-soluble vitamins are best absorbed in oily preparation, such as a gel capsule or drips. Those vitamins are rarely given as injections, and IV administrations need a special form and very specific circumstances, such as parenteral nutrition. Vitamin D is available as an intramuscular injection for nutritional support. Vitamin K is available but indicated to use as an antidote to a blood thinner overdose and not used as a routine supplementation option.

WHAT DEFICIENCIES ARE MOST COMMON AND HOW CAN THEY AFFECT YOU

- Mineral deficiencies are also common in the post-bariatric body. As it's been discussed earlier, iron deficiency is one of the most common side effects of bariatric surgery. There are several more.

- **Calcium deficiency** manifests with facial spasms; muscle cramps; strange sensation in the lips, tongue, and fingers; bone pain; muscular weakness and bone density loss. Calcium utilization is closely connected to sufficient levels of vitamin D and vitamin K. Calcium works in the chemical chain with potassium and magnesium. It is a good idea to check all those minerals and make sure you have optimal levels of them. Fortunately, those minerals are being screened routinely, and most likely, you can find them in your most recent blood work.

- **Trace elements are** minerals present in living tissues in small amounts. The most discussed in this group are zinc, copper, chromium, selenium, manganese, molybdenum, cobalt, and iodine. Of those, zinc and copper deficiencies are well-connected to post-bariatric status. Trace element checking is rarely included during routine blood work, and you need to request this from your health provider if you wish to be checked.

- **Zinc deficiency** manifests as reduced ability to taste things (to taste sweet, sour, bitter, or salty substances); poor appetite; hair loss; muscular weakness; gradually exacerbating eruptions, first affecting the face; nail changes; poor wound healing; depression; poor immunity. Zinc needs to be taken with iron and on an empty stomach. Zinc is also important in the utilization of the thyroid hormone. Prolonged excessive doses may cause toxicity.

- **Copper deficiency** manifests in fragile hair; skin depigmentation; a decrease in white blood cells, red blood cells, and platelets in blood work; muscular weakness; osteoporosis. Copper is potentially toxic and should avoid having an overdose.

- Although is directly investigated in relation to the post-bariatric status, the other trace elements play important role in health.

- **Chromium** takes place in sugar metabolism and is well-known as a factor in weight loss success.

- **Selenium** deficiency causes weakness in the heart muscle, changes in the nails, and suboptimal function of the thyroid hormones.

- **Iodine** is critically important for the normal functioning of the thyroid gland.

EVIDENCE-BASED TEST RECOMMENDATIONS FOR POST- BARIATRIC PATIENTS

- Blood work needs to be done one month after the surgery, then in the 3rd month, 6th month, 12th month, 18th month, 24th month after the date of operation. After two years, blood works needs to be done once a year.

- Bone density test is recommended to be done 12 and 24 months from the date of the surgery. The reason for this test is the high risk for bone demineralization due to all those deficiencies discussed earlier.

- If your blood test shows an elevation in the liver function test, the abdominal ultrasound study is recommended. However, chronic liver conditions, including fatty liver and cirrhosis, tend to improve after bariatric surgery with the progress of weight loss.

- There is a challenge in post-bariatric care. There are no universal standards for bariatric surgical programs during post-surgical follow-ups. After several post-operative visits, you may be referred for future care to your primary care provider. Post-bariatric care is a specific area health expertise, and not all primary care providers are equally familiar with your needs. If you have a choice, choose a primary care provider who works with the post-bariatric population a lot and highly knowledgeable of your needs. You also may consider sharing the information about post-bariatric care with your primary care doctor if needed.

- Well-managed monitoring and correction of deficiencies may significantly improve your surgery results and improve skin quality, hair preservation, and general levels of energy.

REFERENCES

- El-Beheiry M., Vergis A., Choi JU, Clouston K, Hardy K. "A survey of primary care physician referral to Bariatric surgery in Manitoba: access, perceptions and barriers." Supplement 1. Annals Translational Medicine 8 (2020): S3. doi:10.21037/ atm.2020.01.69.

- Levinson, Radmila, Jon B. Silverman, Jennifer G. Catella, Iwona Rybak, Hina Jolin, Kellene. "Isom Pharmacotherapy Prevention and Management of Nutritional Deficiencies Post Roux-en-Y Gastric Bypass." Obesity Surgery 23 (2013): 992–1000. doi:10.1007/s11695-013-0922-2.

- Aron-Wisnewsky, Judith, and Karine Clement. "A place for vitamin supplementation and functional food in bariatric surgery?" Clinical Nutrition and Metabolic Care 22, no. 6 (2019). www.coclinicalnutrition.com.

- Heber, David, Frank L. Greenway, Lee M. Kaplan, Edward Livingston, Javier Salvador, and Christopher Still. "Endocrine and Nutritional Management of the Post-Bariatric Surgery Patient: An Endocrine Society Clinical Practice Guideline." Journal Clinical Endocrinology & Metabolism, 95, no. 11 (2010): 4823–4843. jcem.endojournals.org.

- Busetto, Luca, Dror Dicker, Carmil Azran, Rachel L. Batterham, Nathalie Farpour-Lambert, Martin Fried, Jøran Hjelmesæth, et al. "Practical Recommendations of the Obesity Management Task Force of the European Association for the Study of Obesity for the Post-Bariatric Surgery Medical Management." Obesity Facts 10 (2017): 597-632. doi:10.1159/000481825.

- Jumbe, Sandra, and Jane Meyrick. "Contrasting Views of the Post-Bariatric Surgery Experience between Patients and their Practitioners: A Qualitative Study." Obesity Surgery 28 (2018): 2447–2456. https://doi.org/10.1007/s11695-018-3185-0.

- Gletsu-Miller, Nana,* and Breanne N. Wright. "Mineral Malnutrition Following Bariatric Surgery" Advance Nutrition 4 (2013): 506–517. doi:10.3945/an. 113. 004341.

- Tabesh, Mustang Rajabian, Faezeh Maleklou, Fatemeh Ejtehadi, Zahra Alizadeh. "Nutrition, Physical Activity, and Prescription of Supplements in Pre- and Post-Bariatric Surgery Patients: A Practical Guideline." Obesity Surgery 29 (2019): 3385–3400.

- Agha-Mohammadi, Siamak, B. Chir., Dennis J. Hurwitz. "Nutritional Deficiency of Post–Bariatric Surgery Body Contouring Patients: What Every Plastic Surgeon Should Know." Plastic Reconstruction Surgery 122 (2008): 604.

- Wada, Osamu. "What are Trace Elements? —Their deficiency and excess states." Japan Medical Association Journal 47, no. 8 (2004): 351–358, 2004

EASY GUIDE TO UNDERSTAND IV INFUSIONS

INTRAVENOUS INFUSION (IV) IS A METHOD OF THE ADMINISTRATION OF FLUIDS, MEDICATIONS, OR NUTRIENTS DIRECTLY INTO THE BLOODSTREAM. THE MAJOR ADVANTAGE OF IV THERAPY IS THE BYPASSING OF GASTROINTESTINAL ABSORPTION. IT ELIMINATES THE PROBLEM OF LOSING THE THERAPEUTIC AGENT BEFORE IT GETS INTO THE BLOODSTREAM. IT IS ALSO THE FASTEST AVAILABLE METHOD TO DELIVER FLUIDS AND THERAPEUTIC AGENTS INTO THE BODY.

The most common use of IV infusions is in the treatment of acute illness. IV fluids are given for the treatment of dehydration (loss of water volume in the body); IV antibiotics are the strongest weapon again infections; many other medications are given through IV.

IV is medication considered to be _medically_ necessary if failure to _necessary_ give those medications may lead to the worsening of the person's health condition and is a threat to his/her survival and/or future health status. Medically necessary IVs are the common treatment choice at emergency rooms and hospitals, at the urgent care clinics, and as home care services if the illness so required to prolong therapy.

Over the last several years, there is a popular trend of elective IV infusions (vitamins and minerals) had developed. Those IVs may improve the overall well-being of the recipients but do not have a dramatic impact on the immediate health status.

Medically necessary infusions are usually covered by health insurance. Elective IVs are not covered by insurance.

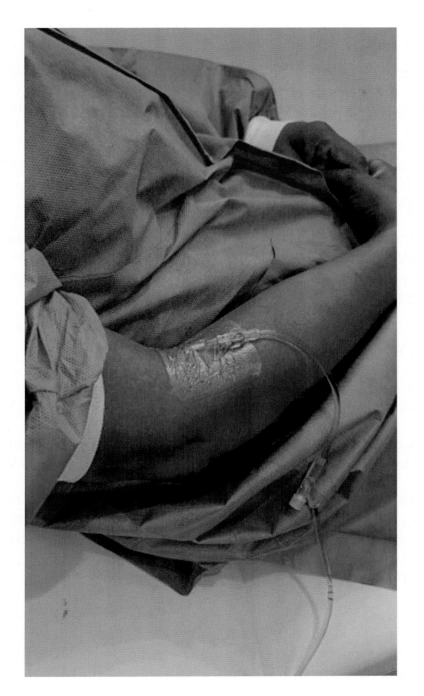

IMPORTANT!

Any IV infusion, would it be medically necessary or elective IV, is a **medical procedure.**

As with any medical procedure, it has benefits but also the potential for complications. To assure proper and safe procedure, the infusion:

1. Must be <u>ordered by a licensed provider</u> with the privilege to prescribe medications (most commonly MD [medical doctor], DO [doctor osteopathy], NP [nurse practitioner], or PA [physician's assistant]).

2. The provider must obtain your medical history. Chronic medical conditions may influence the safety of the infusion. For example, for people with heart failure or kidney problems, an infusion of normal saline may lead to the worsening of a chronic condition if not done with good consideration of the current status.

3. Allergy history must be obtained. It is possible for the infusion to contain ingredients the patient is allergic to.

4. The provider must evaluate your current health status, including vital signs (blood pressure, pulse, respiration, and temperature).

5. The infusion must be done in the proper setting. Emergency equipment must be available. There should be access to emergency services in case of something going wrong.

6. The infusion must be done by a licensed specialist who has the privileges to administer this treatment. Usually, the specialist is a nurse (LPN, RN, APRN or NP), doctor (MD or DO), PA (physician assistant), or EMS. Medical assistants, nurse assistants, venipuncture technicians. or ANY unlicensed paraprofessional personal DO NOT HAVE RIGHTS to administer medications, including IV medication administration.

• Safety complacency is good for most medically necessary IVs. However, the recent trend of elective IV infusions, through which a customer can choose the treatment by IV infusion online or in elective infusion centers, is a concern. For most of the people who decided to get vitamins, IV is preceded by some changes in the health status. Symptoms such as fatigue, pain, poor sleep, hair loss, frequent infections, and more may underline the decision of getting a vitamin infusion. It is a good idea to be evaluated for the origin of those symptoms by your primary care provider before choosing self-treatment options. Those symptoms may be signs of a serious disease, and self-treatment will not resolve those problems but will delay the beginning of the appropriate diagnostic evaluation and therapy.

- Although most ingredients of common elective IV infusions can be found in the vitamin store as a pill, the impact of the same nutrient given through IV is much stronger and may have the potential for adverse reactions that do not occur with an oral form. For example, such a popular ingredient as magnesium given through IV may lead to vasodilation and a drop of blood pressure will result in dizziness and even syncope.

- Common and easy requested supplement, vitamin B12, HAS CONTRAINDICATIONS (cyanocobalamin hypersensitivity, cobalt hypersensitivity, hereditary optic nerve atrophy [Leber's disease] are the examples), and potential for MULTIPLE DRUGS INTERACTIONS. The internet full of poorly reliably, resources, advertising this vitamin for weight loss, energy support, and more. The reality is that none of the vitamins cause weight loss or gain. The healthy levels of vitamin B12 are positive factors during a weight loss program, which includes diet and exercise, but not as an intervention on its own. Fatigue will improve only for the people who have insufficient levels of vitamin B12, but no change will happen if a person has sufficient levels from the beginning. The levels of vitamin B12 can be easily checked during routine blood work.

- Understand, the internet search is a good information resource, but it cannot be considered equal to medical professional advice. Your provider has years of education behind and considering multiple factors. Internet resources do not take any responsibility if you follow advice, and it leads you to problems. Your doctor is responsible, with his/her license, for any advice. <u>Listen to your doctor</u>.

- If you choose to have elective IV, choose a provider who has competency in this area.

- Elective IV therapy HAS CONTRAINDICATIONS! • Absolute: dialysis • relative: chronic renal failure, congestive heart failure, allergy or sensitivity to components, G6PD deficiency, poorly controlled hypertension, seizure disorder, cardiac arrhythmia, nephrolithiasis (kidney stones).

WHEN DO YOU HAVE TO CONSIDER ELECTIVE IV SUPPLEMENTATION

- Ideally, a healthy body gets all nourishment it needs from a healthy diet. If we all would eat high-quality organic, non-GMO food with well-balanced healthy diet choices, most of us would never be deficient in any vitamins or minerals. With corporate agriculture, which exhort the sole, chemical preservatives, toxic components of the food containers, the very methods of food processing and storage many countries used to resolve the problem of starvation at the cost of quality of the food. The same farm produce and grains, which were nutritionally sufficient a century ago, may have fewer vitamins and minerals. However, the deficiencies often can be managed with oral supplementation of vitamins and minerals.

- The need for IV infusions (or muscular and subdermal injections) comes when the gastrointestinal tract cannot normally absorb the nutrients supplied. This condition is called malabsorption. Conditions which may cause malabsorption are the following:

- <u>Chronic gastritis, duodenitis, colitis, IBS syndrome, Crohn's disease</u> (or some other gastrointestinal conditions the affect absorption).

- <u>Long-term use of PPI</u> (proton pump inhibitors), a medication group often prescribed for gastritis and gastric reflux disease. Esomeprazole [Nexium], lansoprazole [Prevacid], omeprazole [Prilosec] are the examples of medications of this group).

- <u>Surgeries</u> with partial removal of the stomach or intestine, such as bariatric surgeries (surgeries that are done to treat obesity), all types of GI tumor–related surgeries, intestinal obstruction surgeries, and more.

- <u>Chronic medical conditions</u>, such as diabetes, may affect absorption.

- <u>Long-term use of anti-inflammatory medications</u>, both nonsteroidal (ibuprofen/brand names Motrin and Advil, Naproxen, Celecoxib/brand name Celebrex, meloxicam/brand name Mobic are the examples) and steroid type (prednisone, dexamethasone, many asthma pumps that contain steroids are the examples) may affect GI absorption.

- <u>Alcoholism</u>, among other things, affects intestinal absorption.

Those are the most common causes of malabsorption, but certainly, there are many more. If those factors are present, oral supplementation of minerals and vitamins may not be enough.

Elective IVs preparation can be done in the compounding pharmacy or in the clinic by an eligible provider.

Both options have cons and pros.

An IV kit prepared by a compounding pharmacy is usually preordered; the pharmacy has tested this compound for stability before offering it to the doctors. The preparation is done in a well-controlled sterile setting.

If the compound is mixed in the clinic, your provider has more flexibility to adjust the preparation to a patient's individual needs and current health condition. It requires a higher level of expertise but can be more effective.

Higher levels of elective IVs are usually offered at the clinics specializing in functional, regenerative, or anti-aging medicine. Although those specialties are still not recognized at the same level as, let say cardiology or endocrinology, there are professional organizations dedicated to the development of this line of knowledge. They promote medical research on the related subject and educates health care professionals who are looking to develop competency in those areas of expertise. They are also offering board examination can search for providers-members of those organizations and board-certified providers in your area on the website of these organizations:

American Academy of Anti-Aging Medicine https://www.a4m.com/

American Academy of Functional Medicine https://americanacademyoffunctionalmedicine.org

The Institute for Functional Medicine https://www.ifm.org

OVERVIEW OF MOST COMMON ELECTIVE IVS:

- Myer's cocktail is probably the most common elective IV infusion. This formulation is based on the clinical development of Dr. John Myer, who lived and practiced in Baltimore during the 1960s and1970s and died in1984. He used this preparation to treat many conditions, including chronic fatigue, asthma, migraines, acute respiratory infections, and more. Dr. Myer did not document the exact prescription, and all current information is based on the article published in 2002 by Dr. Alan Gaby. Dr. Gaby recovered the original formula as much as it was possible due to the lack of official documentation by interviewing former patients of Dr. Myer and adjusting the formula according to his best judgment of safety and stability. Dr. Gaby's formula consists of a mix of magnesium chloride, calcium gluconate, vitamin B12, vitamin B6, vitamin B5, B-complex, and vitamin C. Dr. Gaby's formula is what we now use as the Myer's cocktail standard.

Some practitioners considered adjusting this formula by adding some additional ingredients or changing the proportion based on the clinical situation of the patient.

- The research data about the effectiveness of the Myer's cocktail is controversial, but there is a very good number of patients and clinicians who favored its benefits.

- Common **indications** for Myer's cocktails are: • asthma • migraines • chronic fatigue syndrome • fibromyalgia • muscle spasm • coronary artery disease • upper respiratory infections • chronic sinusitis • and allergic rhinitis

- Hangover IV is used for treating acute alcoholic intoxication. It is good medical advice to not consume alcohol at the amount that may require medical help for recovery. However, if the situation went out of control, IV fluids alone may be useful for hydration

(alcohol dehydrates the body), increase toxin excretion, and protect the liver and kidney from the

poisonous effect of alcohol. Besides the fluids, vitamin B complex, vitamin B1 (thiamin), and vitamin B6 (pyroxene) are often added to the infusion to support the liver. Amino acid taurine is also included in the hangover formulas.

- Hydrogen Peroxide IV infusions are a less common infusion but still can be useful in the right circumstances. This infusion can be potentially dangerous if not administrated correctly. Make sure you have been treated by a qualified provider if you are getting it. Hydrogen peroxide infused alone should not be combined with any other infusions.

Indications: • COPD • chronic asthma • bronchitis • fungemia • acute URI • viral infections

Hydrogen peroxide infusion can also be used as a choice for *oxidative therapy* (to increase blood and tissue oxygenation) in the conditions of infections, viral and bacterial (acute/chronic) • fatigue • Lyme syndromes, CFS, FM • allergies, sensitivities to chemicals • arthritis • autoimmune diseases • chronic pain.

- Glutathione is a substance naturally produced by the liver but also found in plants. It is one of the most powerful antioxidants (the substances that can prevent or slow damage to cells caused by free radicals and unstable molecule). Glutathione has multiple uses: detoxification, support normal functioning of nerve cells, anti-inflammatory, and more. Glutathione is available in an oral preparation, inhalation but more effective if given IV. Indications: "Failure to detoxify" • autoimmune diseases, including Lyme • chronic inflammation • liver, gut (SIBO), kidney disease • toxic metal syndrome • neurogenic inflammation—brain fog, MS, dementia, PD, neuropathies, "chemo brain." Glutathione is a very safe infusion and works best if given in combination with Myer's cocktail. Glutathione is a useful tool for the management of neurodegenerative diseases, such as Alzheimer's and Parkinson's. Although it is most surely not a cure, it does improve the functional status of the patient. It can be used for the treatment of acute intoxication, including alcoholic intoxication. Studies using intravenous glutathione have found it to be useful for reducing the side effects and increasing the efficacy of chemotherapy drugs.

- **Precautions**: rapid infusion can provoke respiratory distress, coughing, rhinorrhea ("runny nose"), and vertigo (dizziness).

- **Common clinical outcome**: increased energy, improved memory.

- **High-dose vitamin C infusions** are infusions of vitamin C in doses between 15 and 100gm. Although vitamin C is included in some IV compounds (Myer's cocktail is an example), it's usually used in much lesser dose.

- **Low-dose IVC** is in between 0.07 to 0.14 grams per kilogram of body weight. This concentration is used for general immune and antioxidant support; occasionally is given with glutathione.

- **High-dose oxidative IV vitamin C** is 0.4 to 1.4 grams per kilogram of body weight. Those doses are for purely oxidative purposes and generally only have minerals to balance blood electrolytes, such as magnesium, calcium, and potassium, and are not given with glutathione or other nutrients and antioxidants on the same day. High-dose vitamin C infusion has the potential for causing metabolic and electrolyte changes and can be dangerous if not given correctly. Must be done by a qualified provider in the clinical setting. Infusion time is dosage-dependent, may take between 30 minutes to 2.5 hours. A laboratory test is recommended prior to high-dose vitamin C infusion therapy: CBC and G6PD testing. There is a record of fatality with high-dose vitamin C infusion when those precautions were not done.

- **Indications for <u>oxidative therapy</u>**: infections, viral and bacterial (acute/chronic) • fatigue • Lyme syndromes • allergies, sensitivities to chemicals • arthritis • autoimmune diseases • chronic pain.

- IV use of vitamin C actively discussed is as an adjunct treatment of cancer. There is a study showing a high concentration of Vitamin C (only achievable through IV administration) <u>has tumor-inhibiting activities.</u>

There is a protocol for the use of vitamin C infusions in combination with chemotherapy, recommending the use of the infusion of vitamin C the same day with chemotherapy before administrating the chemotherapy agent. Glutathione and high-dose vitamin C concur with each other when used as an adjunct to chemotherapy. Only one agent should be chosen.

- Chelation is a therapy that cleans the body of toxic metals. Chelation is used in conventional medicine to treat acute heavy metals poisoning. Acute metal poisoning is a serious medical condition that is usually treated in the hospital.

- Functional medicine providers are more focused on chronic heavy metal poisoning that may develop over years and years through exposure to low-dose environmental toxins and may not be recognized as a state of disease by traditional medical providers. A functional medical provider sees chronic metal intoxication as one of the main causes of chronic inflammation, which leads to many chronic diseases, the most common of which is cardiovascular disease and neurodegenerative disease.

- Chelation therapy is done by administrating chelation agents, EDTA and DMSA. Among conditions which may benefit from chelation therapy, the functional medicine provider recognizes: • CAD/CVD • PAD • post-MI, post-stroke • microvascular disease • hypertension • hyperlipidemia • toxic metal syndrome • MCS • Lyme syndrome.

- Although there are research and clinical data that support the functional medicine approach, chelation therapy is certainly is not a treatment that can be done without special training. The chelation regiment is highly specific and individual, requires lab work up to before treatment. Dosage calculation is patient-specific and takes into account renal function, gender, patient weight, and more. Because of advances, the expertise required for this type of therapy, the author of this guide recommends considering the treatment only under the supervision of a medical doctor in the clinic well-equipped to

- Magnesium is a component of many wellness IV mixes. Magnesium is one of the most important minerals in our body. Magnesium plays a role in the energy production, structuring of the bones, needed for the cell signaling—nerve impulses, muscular construction, relaxation of blood vessels, the electrical activity of the heart, and more. Magnesium is a part of Myer's cocktail.

- In combinations with L-arginine and vitamin B6, it is used for the treatment of high blood pressure.

- In combination with L-arginine, vitamin C, vitamins B6 and B12, it is used to treat acute asthma.

- Used for the treatment of migraine.

- Use for the treatment of chronic muscular pain and spasms.

- Included in the immunocapture combination drips and rehydration mix.

- Alpha-lipoic acid (ALA) is an antioxidant, the most known of its benefits is blood glucose control. The other uses of ALA infusion are for chronic fatigue • diabetes • liver disease • autoimmune disease • heavy metal toxicity • MCS • cancer • peripheral neuropathy.

ALA is to be infused along with, and this infusion also needs to be administered slowly over several hours.

Curcumin is a very powerful antioxidant, often used in oral forms for the treatment of inflammation and joint pain. IV curcumin has been yet another infusion that must be done in the appropriate clinical environment. There is a record of a severe, life-threatening allergic reaction to this compound. No other component can be mixed in the IV bag with curcumin.

NAD + (nicotinamide adenine dinucleotide) is a well-known supplement that supports the prevention of premature skin aging, Alzheimer's disease management, diabetes, heart disease, and vision loss. The original use of IV NAD is for the treatment of drug addiction. IV NAD+ is very effective and gives almost immediate effect. The dark side of this infusion is that it is to be given slowly and is often associated with transitional but noticeable discomfort.

Resveratrol is a substance found in many plants. There are many studies confirming Resveratrol has antitumor potential, but also, it is anti-inflammatory, anticarcinogenic, cardioprotective, vasorelaxant, phytoestrogenic, and neuroprotective. This infusion is less commonly offered, possibly due to the fact that it still remains challenging to find supplies and the cost of infusion. However, for the right use, it is a powerful and strong tool.

REFERENCES

- "Cyanocobalamin - Drug Summary." PDR Prescriber's Digital References. https://www.pdr.net/drug- summary/Nascobal-cyanocobalamin-2286#10

- Gallagher, Martin, and Emma McGowan. "IV, IM & Oral Nutritional Therapy in Regenerative." (Dallas, Texas, 2018), 19–20.

- Gaby, Alan R. "Intravenous Nutrient Therapy: the 'Myers' Cocktail.'" Alternative Medicine Review 7, no. 5 (2002): 389–403.

- Perry TL et al. "Ideopathic Parkinson's disease: A disorder due to nigra glutathione deficiency." Neuroscience Letter 67 (1986): 269–274.

- Sechi, G. et al. "Reduced intravenous glutathione in the treatment of early Parkinson's disease." Progress in Neuro-Psychopharmacology & Biological Psychiatry 20 (1996):1159–1170.

- Johnson WM, et al. "Dysregulation of glutathione homeostasis in neurodegenerative diseases." Nutrients. 4, no. 10 (2012): 1399–1440. doi:10.3390/nu4101399.

- Hotamisligil G.S. "Inflammation and metabolic disorders." Nature. 444:860-867 2006

- Herder C., Illig T., Rathmann W. "Inflammation and type 2 diabetes: results from KORA Augsburg." Supplement 1. Gesundheitswesen 67 (2005): S115–S121.

- Livshits Z., Hoffman RS, Hymes KB, Nelson LS. "If vitamins could kill: massive hemolysis following naturopa this vitamin infusion." Journal of Medical Toxicology 7, no. 3 (2011): 224–226.

- Salehi, Bahare, Abhay Prakash Mishra, Manisha Nigam, Bilge Sener, Mehtap Kilic, Mehdi Sharifi- Rad 6,

- Patrick Valere South Fokou et al. "Resveratrol: A Double-Edged Sword." Health Biomedicines 6 (2018): 91.

Printed in the United States
by Baker & Taylor Publisher Services